DEDICATION

This book is dedicated to my dad and the other courageous souls battling dementia and to my mom and the other everyday heroes who are taking care of them.

KEEP GIVING A CARE:
THE CONCISE GUIDE FOR ALZHEIMER'S AND OTHER DEMENTIA FAMILY CAREGIVERS

PRATIBHA VANMALI

CONTENTS

ACKNOWLEDGMENTS

With immeasurable love and respect, I thank my mother, Madhuben. She is both the gentlest and the strongest person I know. Her inimitable gentle strength, her wisdom, and her loving heart have been saving graces in our family's dementia journey and throughout my life.

This book could not have been written without the support and love of my husband, Michael. I offer him deep gratitude for helping with the editing process, being my rock throughout the writing process, and steadfastly helping me help my family through these caregiving years.

Last but not least, I thank my sister, Binaben, and my dog, Lotus. My sister was the first person to recognize, then critique to cultivate, my writing talent at an early age. Her guidance and push have been significant driving forces behind my writing endeavors. Lotus has unwaveringly been by my side as I've typed, cried, laughed, and revised my way through this book. Her emotional support is invaluable, as are her reminders to give myself a break for some fresh air and sunshine.

INTRODUCTION

"Life is worth living as long as there's a laugh in it."
Lucy Maud Montgomery

Some people know from an early age exactly what they want to be when they "grow up." I'm not one of those people. Maybe I'm not grown up yet. As a child, I had a variety of career aspirations, and as an adult, I've been blessed to have successfully explored and fulfilled most of them. However, one title that was not on the list was "caregiver." But perhaps it is the most important one.

It's also one in which I find I'm constantly learning new lessons about my family, about the way the world works, about the way the world doesn't work for those dealing with dementia, and about myself. In this book, I'll share some of those lessons and effective strategies to navigate them in hopes of making your caregiving journey a little lighter and helping you feel less alone in it. To this end, I understand how difficult carving out time for yourself, including to read a book, can be while caring for someone with Alzheimer's Disease and/or other forms of dementia. With this in mind, I've written this book to be comprehensive without being superfluous.

In your journey, you're going to have many humbling moments that take different shapes. As such, the tone of this book is multidimensional, adding humor to humility. And as a caregiver to someone with dementia, you know or will soon come to understand just how important tone is. With this said, parts of this book might come off as flippant or unloving. But to clarify, I never aim to be unloving. However, flippant may indeed be the intention at times; because in reality, we are all human. And sometimes as a caregiving human, your only options are either to be crushed by reality or to have a laugh at it.

CHAPTER 1:
THIS TIME MACHINE IS WARPED

"God, grant me the serenity to accept the things I cannot change; courage to change the things I can; and wisdom to know the difference."
Reinhold Niebuhr

One of the many dreams I had in childhood was to become a real estate agent. I'd even set up fort and give tours. And the really hot properties would bring bidding wars between the teddy bears and the dolls.

Many years later, after I'd become a real estate agent, there came a time that I'd relocated to a new area and was getting to know my new broker. Unbeknownst to her, two years prior to that move, my dad had been diagnosed with dementia. At the time of my move, he was still functioning more or less like he always had, so I hadn't fully grasped what this diagnosis would bring.

So when my new broker spoke of moving her mother who had Alzheimer's Disease across the country to take better care of her, I silently wondered if my larger-than-life dad would ever need or accept that type of assistance. And when she joked about this disease allowing her to see what her mom was like as a child, I found that thought to be almost heartwarming. I didn't know then that one day I would understand that her little chuckle in that moment was actually masking a heavy sadness.

Becoming the parent of your parent in ways that make you laugh, scream, and cry (sometimes all at once), was never on the list of any of our childhood dreams. And going from the trenches of imaginary and actual bidding wars of real estate to the all-to-real trenches of caregiving, I now know that seeing and protecting your parent as they were in childhood can both break and warm the heart. This most recent Mother's Day, I received a text message from a friend that spoke directly to this task and sentiment. It read, "The tender love and care you show for your parents is much like a mother's love. So, I'll wish you a happy Mother's Day." That love and committed care she spoke of resonated very deeply, but in my reply, I jokingly blamed the tears that it brought to my eyes on my menstrual cycle.

Having traveled a decade into the darkness of this disease, I don't specifically remember the very first time the thought of my parent reverting to childlike behaviors resonated with me. However, I am pretty sure that the instance it could no longer be denied surrounded a new dining habit that would be unconventional in any culture and at any age. Over time, my dad had started eating lunch out of smaller and smaller plates. He continued this until he eventually decided that plates were both unnecessary and inadequate in catching the crumbs of his margarine and potato chip sandwiches. After coming to that conclusion, he'd try to eat them on newspaper. And to put it into complete context, it's important to note that these were sandwiches he'd insist on making with about half an inch of margarine coating the insides of both pieces of bread and with the potato chips in between. They were not sandwiches which featured margarine as the condiment and potato chips on the side. Looking back, I suppose he might have created the most efficient way to eat a sandwich with chips. And I think he'd take some pride in that, since until dementia slowed him down, he tackled almost every task with a speed of someone trying to outrun a cheetah and winning productivity awards throughout his career. Beyond having bizarre cravings and an eventually decreased appetite, your loved one may also start resisting or refusing to use eating utensils. This is because they may be experiencing sensory and cognitive impairment, which can cause difficulty figuring out how to use utensils. Offering weighted cutlery with large handles or allowing them to eat with their hands can be helpful in assisting your loved one with continuing to be able to eat with a sense of independence without feeling embarrassed.

Regardless of not pinning down the exact moment in time when I first found myself reflecting on the realization that I was seeing my parent as he was in childhood, I am certain of how disheartened I felt when it did click and how surprised I was at my dad's petulant reaction to my pushback on his altered behavior. I felt sadness. I felt anger. I also felt fear. Seeing my dad acting so often in such nonsensical and embarrassing ways was incredibly sad. I was angry that as an adult, he was stubbornly doubling down on his childish behavior, and it baffled me that he didn't understand why I was upset about it. And frankly, I was scared of what the future was going to bring if this past was becoming our present.

But after I'd had time and space to process (which came after several more contentious encounters), I surprisingly also felt a helpful shift in my mindset. I realized that he usually wasn't meaning to upset me by acting like a child. This seemingly small realization has brought me a relatively large degree of peace many times over these caregiving years. As such, that instance and countless situations since then have taught and reminded me that rather than trying to correct him into acting like the adult I see before me, I need to accept that he sees things differently now. Therefore, it's imperative that I see him differently. I have to perceive and receive him as who he is now, which in many ways is who he was as a kid but not who he was when I was a kid. This is not easy to reconcile, but I've absolutely needed to adjust my behavior accordingly, because he can't.

Peeking back in time like this, I've come to a rather solid conclusion that he was a spoiled and bratty child. I've also come to a place where I can approach these time-machine moments with more than just futile resistance, frustration, and anger. Not every conventional victory is worth the win. When his child-like actions aren't harmful or likely to have lasting impact, I now aim to handle these situations with greater acceptance and by taking a loss that's sometimes accompanied with a laugh. And in the occasional moments that he joins me in that laughter, it's actually a win.

CHAPTER 2:
I CAN'T BELIEVE MY EYES

"There are things known and there are things unknown, and in between are the doors of perception."
Aldous Huxley

"Gas!" my father loudly yelled at nobody within earshot who could help. This happened on a nice afternoon in which I'd ridden with my dad to the gas station. I was enjoying the sensation of the warm sunshine streaming through the window as I waited in his vehicle while he got fuel. I contentedly sat there until the pleasant early summer sounds of birds chirping was interrupted by him screaming this one word towards the convenience store. He had not hit the help button. The clerk did not hear him, but the many customers who were outside did. Their stares of disbelief were palpable.

Upon my jumping out of the vehicle to see what was going on, he expressed great frustration about the pump. He said it was not working. I didn't understand why my father, the man who had taught me how to drive, suddenly couldn't get a fuel pump that he'd used many times before to work, nor why he thought that screaming would be the fix and a socially acceptable one at that. Regardless, I showed him how to do it. With that, he filled up, and we left the confused and shocked onlookers behind.

In that instance, the concerns my sister had recently been voicing to me about his extra-erratic behavior came to life in a way that could only be seen as embarrassing at the time, but that I can now look back on and find funny. He was diagnosed with dementia within a year or so after this incident.

Leading up to this, my sister, who was living with my parents at the time, called me to discuss a dramatically strange shift in Dad's behavior. My dad has always marched to the beat of his own drum. But it seemed that his drum was now out of tune.

He had smoked cigarettes during his rebellious teenage years and drank alcohol as a young adult, but he has never done drugs. However, when my sister and I were discussing his current behavior and this recent incident, with dementia not being on either of our radars, we seriously wondered if our dad had started taking drugs. His job required him to travel into various areas and interact with people from many walks of life. So although it didn't seem likely that he was on drugs, it did seem like a plausible scenario that we needed to look into.

With this, we hatched a master plan to figure out who his dealer was and to set my dad back on track. Simple. And safe, right? Looking back, I can see so many holes in our strategy. But at least it started strong: with a spreadsheet.

My sister sent me a list of his mobile call log. From there, I created a spreadsheet and called every single number that I didn't recognize, making detailed notes with each attempt. I did this with a rather ignorant courage, ready to question whoever would answer. My sister was amazed at how boldly I was proceeding. I did not get anywhere with this. But perhaps it's for the best that I didn't reach and confront an actual drug dealer.

Nowadays, we don't go through his phone logs. Now we understand that he was not and is not on drugs, but that he has lost his way in a very different way. He doesn't actually physically get lost yet, but we know that is a real possibility to come and one for which we need to try to be prepared. To keep him safe during the infrequent occasions that he is unaccompanied or in the case that he should ever wander unexpectedly, we've explored a few different covert options.

Thus far, we've tried GPS tile trackers that can go in pockets, connect to pet collars, or be attached to keychains, the Life360 app, and location tracking on his phone. Each of these has helped, but none have been a perfect solution for our family. But it's important to keep in mind that each patient and family are different, so one or all of these might be the right fit for your situation.

We found the GPS tile trackers to be effective, but their main drawback was the relatively small radius that they'd cover. Now that Dad doesn't enjoy walks, especially long walks, these might be worth revisiting for him or for your loved one who doesn't regularly tend to venture far from home.

Life360 and location tracking on his phone did solve the radius issue. However, they weren't equipped, and honestly neither are we some days, to tackle the issue of his stubborn noncompliance. They will only work in real-time if the person keeps the device with them and turned on. However, with phone location tracking, the service provider can show the last known location once the phone is switched back on. And they both do offer location history covering differing timeframes which could be useful in locating a lost loved one, especially in lengthy search situations.

There are several options available for dementia patients who are more willing to utilize them. A couple of these include alert patches with alarms and GPS watches. My dad currently refuses to wear those or any others. I've also created a simpler safety measure. It's a card that identifies your loved one and that they have dementia, and it notes an emergency contact. I have included it at the end of this book for your loved one to carry in a wallet, pocket, or purse.

Another option is an air tracker tag which can be more easily disguised. As such, we are looking at air trackers that can be hidden in special soles that would go in my dad's favorite walking shoes. If he refuses the soles, then we will be back at square one.

Square one is a place that you'll revisit many times on this caregiving journey. It's not a comfortable place, but it's instead an overly welcoming one in which you might sometimes feel like you're held hostage. I have realized however, that square one actually becomes a less foreign place with each visit on the same matter. This is important because searching for a solution becomes less elusive with each failed attempt. While each option that doesn't work can bring disheartenment and frustration, it helps to remember that knowing what isn't working is guiding you closer to what will. And this discernment is profound when you're feeling the weight of a seemingly unsolvable problem.

Since many people with dementia do wander, a simple option to deter this, which doesn't require tools to install, is to tie bells, such as jingle bells, on the door knobs to create an alert sound. It's also recommended to install deadbolts and doorknob covers or grips to help avoid the possibility of your loved one leaving the house without notice and getting lost. And it's useful to place additional locks away from their normal range of vision.

Vision is a fluid concept that goes beyond the literal when it comes to dementia. My sister and I saw my father's behaviors at the very early onset as outlandish enough to send us on a humorously wild goose chase. My dad increasingly sees the world through the eyes of a child, but with the indignation of an adult. Ultimately, it stands to reason that none of our individual ways of seeing the moment would be considered 20/20.

CHAPTER 3:
NOT NORMAL

At some point during adolescence, it's normal for many kids to find at least one of their parents embarrassing. Some parents embrace this stage by having fun with it. The father of one of my elementary school friends was known to plot on her slumber parties in an effort to purposely embarrass her in front of her friends. His attempts were successful because she'd be humiliated, and we'd be entertained. Some parents ignore this stage and others resist it by forcing hugs at the school drop-off line. And eventually, most children become young adults who outgrow that feeling, and the embarrassment is replaced with intrigue and a newfound respect.

My dad has always remained eccentric in an authentic way, regardless of how I, or of how I have thought the world, perceived him. Once dementia took hold, his eccentricities multiplied and showed out in new and intentionally noticeable ways.

For example, we were dining out one night at a nice establishment. This was a special evening since our whole family was together, which hadn't happened in many years, as my sister had moved to Arizona by then. Luckily, I knew the owners of this restaurant and had advised them of my dad's condition before our arrival. They seemed understanding and welcoming. But even with this prior knowledge, they, just like their other restaurant guests, seemed shocked and nervous when Dad got up and loudly proclaimed that he was cold, made a production out of putting on his coat, and started walking around the quaint and otherwise quiet dining area.

A couple of years later, as my parents and I were about to walk into our first Alzheimer's Support Group meeting, I was also experiencing another first. It was a feeling that I hope you have found or will find along your caregiving journey. In that moment, I felt sweet relief. This relief was the weight of others' judgement about my dad's behavior being lifted. I realized that it was the first time since his diagnosis and progression that I would be amongst strangers who'd intimately understand any oddities or offenses in my dad's words or actions. When I shared this thought with my mom, I could see that cloud of worry clearing from her eyes, too. Even though COVID put an end to those meetings, those strangers have now become friends who mutually understand the normality in this abnormal journey, friends with which embarrassment around demented behaviors doesn't exist.

These support group meetings have been valuable beyond offering a priceless community of understanding. They've also provided information, resources, and glimmers of hope in what sometimes feels like a hopeless journey.

One of the resources they gave us came in the compact size of a business card. It was a card sized to fit in a wallet or pocket and designed to let someone know that your companion has dementia and to thus ask the other party for patience. When I first got it, I didn't know how soon I'd need it or if I would ever have the courage to show it.

That day came sooner than I'd expected. It was about a year and a half after our first support group meeting. I'd taken my parents to their vision exams, during the stage where my dad found it hilarious to joke about being hit with a sledgehammer. My dad likes to joke around and people have generally found him to be funny over his lifetime.

However, most people who'd hear this icebreaking joke about sledgehammers would just politely give a confused giggle. The receptionists at this office found zero humor in it, not even cracking a smile. Consequently, he kept repeating the joke in different ways. I suppose he was thinking that they didn't hear him or really get it, and once they did, that they would crack up just as much as him. I could see that they did hear it, but that they neither got it, nor appreciated it. In an effort to tamp down their irritation, I collected my dad (redirecting him to try on frames) and then collected my courage to pull that card out of my wallet and actually show it to someone. It was a scary and magical moment. When I saw the instant shifts in their annoyed countenance to one of patience, resulting in warm smiles directed at my mom and me and a kinder approach with my dad, the anxiety dissipated and that newly discovered feeling of relief returned to me. Since then, I've used the card a handful of times. But now I use it without embarrassment or hesitation and with the expectation of a level of empathy. Thankfully, it has delivered that humanity each time. I've included a similar card for you at the end of this book.

Another tool that we've found to be useful is the Alzheimer's Association Caregiver Helpline which can be reached at +1-800-272-3900, twenty-four hours a day, seven days a week. It's a confidential resource in which you can talk to a dementia expert for support, crisis assistance, information about virtual and online support groups and other resources, and it's available in over 200 languages. It's also a place that on the other end of the line, you are offered hope as you're met with that relief of an understanding voice.

CHAPTER 4:
NEIGHBORHOOD WATCH

"A little among neighbors is worth more than riches in a wilderness."
Welsh Proverb

Sometimes keeping my peace in this journey has meant letting go of discovering details that I might've otherwise inquired about before this caregiving chapter of life started. For example, a neighbor who is friendly, but who is not a close friend, recently made a point of interrupting her family dinner on their deck to catch me on my walk to ask how I was doing and to offer an ear or shoulder to cry on.

Why? My dad had recently visited with her when he was on a walk. Something about their interaction prompted her to extend this kind offer of support to me, telling me that her door is always open and that she's praying for my family. Since this went beyond our usual small talk, I would've, in the past, asked what happened during their conversation; but that evening, I decided to let their chat be theirs and to just feel satisfied in knowing she said that he's sweet (versus problematic) and to feel a peace and gratitude in her offer of support.

While I cannot, and am learning should not, keep a watchful eye on every small matter, keeping my dad safe is a top priority. To this end, I'm thankful for her and for other neighbors who have helped me keep a watchful eye.

The first time my sister was diagnosed with cancer and my mom went to Arizona to help her, my husband and I took over full-time caregiving of my dad. Since he was staying with us during this time, I, as a precaution, had let a couple of neighbors know that he has dementia should his jokes or behaviors raise eyebrows. Or worse, should he have gotten lost.

One evening before sunset, he went for a walk. I was aware he'd wanted to go, so I set up the location tracking link on his phone and asked him to keep his phone turned on. During his walk, one of those neighbors I'd informed about his condition, texted me to ask if I knew he was on a walk and to see if he was okay. I thanked her and confirmed that I was aware of his walk and whereabouts and that he had just safely made it home. Since the tone of her text had alluded to a potential problem, I asked my dad if he was okay or if he had encountered any problems on his walk. He said he was fine and that nothing out of the ordinary had happened.

A few weeks later when I was on a walk, I spoke with her husband who working outside in his yard. Since his retirement, I often see him outside and catch up with him while our dogs catch up with each other. When he brought up my dad's walk, he said that some kids he hadn't seen before were following my dad and harassing him about his age. He noted the one who was the biggest bully in stature and in personality seemed especially loud and intent on the chase. But the big bully ran off when my neighbor called them out on their behavior. My neighbor was hoping to tell him to stop and to ask where he lived so that he could talk to the boy's parents about his inappropriate behavior. One of the younger ones stayed and talked with my neighbor, and he sternly instructed her that they should never again follow or bother my dad.

He said my dad didn't seem phased by them. This element was both comforting and concerning, but it helped to make sense of why Dad hadn't mentioned it to me. Overall, I felt extremely grateful for my neighbor's intervention and glad that neither he, nor my dad, were hurt. This also made me realize how important it was to learn where another neighbor who has told me he has dementia lives. In the past three years of our chats during his evening strolls, I've noticed a decline in his cognition. As such, knowing his address could be lifesaving should his walks ever land him in trouble or at a place from which he doesn't know how to get home.

The year before my dad came to stay with us, I'd informed a couple of my parents' neighbors about his condition. I had not informed the neighbor upon whose property line and theirs housed a mobility scooter that had been lying in the same spot for a couple of months. I didn't know much about mobility scooters, but I did know that one didn't belong in their front yard, even if it was somewhat hidden behind a bush. As my dad's dementia has progressed, my dad's tendency to go what I'll call treasure hunting and stash his finds has also increased. So I asked him about it. He said it belonged to the neighbor. So when I saw her outside shortly after he told me that, I asked her if she needed help moving it. She said it wasn't theirs and thought it was Dad's because she'd seen him working on it.

That information made my blood boil to the point of matching the temperature of that hot summer day. He not only didn't need that scooter, but he also lied straight to my face about it. I was becoming accustomed and almost numb to his lies that were becoming so outrageous at times that all I could do was laugh at them. But my actions after hearing the truth about this scooter that was just lying there killing the grass (that my dad wouldn't stop digging up), showed that I wasn't immune to his lies or the disrespect I felt in being lied to like that.

You'll notice that as this disease progresses, the person you're caring for will become a storyteller. If they already were a teller of tales, then they'll become a bigger one. This doesn't equate to a better one because there will be times that you'll feel like they are doubting your intelligence with the unbelievable stories they'll fabricate. At times, grace should be given since their lies might be covering up something they're uncertain about. I felt like this, which was a blatant lie, was not one of those times, and I could not let it roll of my shoulders. What ensued was me ensnaring myself in the tangled web my dad had weaved!

With Dad inside, I made it my immediate mission to get rid of that scooter. Until then, I had had no idea how heavy that thing was. But I pulled on, grunted at, cursed at, and pushed it out of their yard and down the sidewalk toward the car. I was not getting far or going fast, but I was determined to get it in their trunk to dispose of it. During this ignominious scene, a car passed by whose driver waved at me. Since I didn't live there, I didn't know who it was, but I gave a wave back, wiped the sweat out of my eyes, and got back to the task at hand. Then I saw one of the other neighbors who I'd told about my dad's dementia get out of that car and walk over.

What an embarrassing relief! It was clear that while he wasn't sure exactly what he was about to walk up to, he knew that I looked like I needed help. With that, he carried it down the sidewalk and helped me get it into their trunk, with the understanding that I would never tell my dad that he was involved. We did not want World War III to break out over this broken-down equipment that had at this point almost broken me down, emotionally and physically.

I told my mom what was going on, and that evening, we got permission to dispose of it in a friend's business' dumpster. We went after they closed. With nobody there but us, I summoned all the rage I had within me to lift it, but I could not safely get it out of their car.

Hours into this fiasco, with the success of the mission now hanging by a thread, we drove back to my parents' house with the scooter still in tow. I told my dad that the utility service men who happened to be working in the area at the time said it was in their way and helped me get it into their trunk. Yes, now I was lying to him. He agreed to help me get it out of their trunk and onto the curb. Once again at square one, I decided to see if it had any kind of indicator on it. It did! The next morning, I called the company whose name was on the plaque, and while they didn't know who it belonged to, they sent somebody to collect it, hoping that replacing its battery could put it back in service.

I don't know what the conversation between my neighbor across the street and my dad entailed, why those kids were picking on my dad, or if the scooter's battery was salvageable or not. But I do know that in this caregiving journey, helping and accepting help from neighbors is at times a necessity in keeping our batteries charged and our loved ones safe.

CHAPTER 5:
MIXED SIGNALS

*"Personality has power to uplift, power to depress, power to curse,
and power to bless."*
Paul P. Harris

He just stood there staring at her. As I walked into my parents' dining room, I saw my dog urgently doing her pee pee dance by the patio door. My dad, who was positioned the closest to her, was standing there, just staring at her. When I alerted him to the fact that she needed out and asked him to open the door, he said with irritation, "I know. That's what I'm doing." Later in the day, their dog, who like my father, also suffers from cognitive decline, thought she was stuck in a corner. So I asked my dad to help her since he was right next to her. His response was, "I know. I'm going to do it." Again, he sounded irritated even though there's no question that he loves our dogs. Thus, the irritation was seemingly directed at me. Since the words, "I know," are clear and concise, and usually meant to send a direct message, you can imagine the irritation I was feeling hearing them without action to match.

But what I've actually come to know is that when these words are spoken by people afflicted with dementia, they are many times coming from a cloudy place in the mind that's actually thinking, "I should have known," or "Okay." Thus, the irritation accompanying the, "I know," is likely directed internally. And knowing this can help ease irritation for both you as the caregiver and for your loved one with dementia.

Beyond loving our dogs, my dad loves music and movies. His affinity runs so deep for each of these things that he played in a band in his youth, later worked in the film industry, and has publicly sung at important family events as a senior citizen. So I didn't understand as his responses to invitations for going to the movies or to watch live music performances changed from the once enthusiastic, "Yes," to the tentative "Maybe," and then ultimately to the definitive, "No." The only thing is, the, "No," is not as certain as the intonation in his voice makes it sound.

This assertive, "No," often actually translates to, "I don't know." What he doesn't know is either what he's being asked to partake in or if it's a situation in which he'll feel safe or comfortable. This, although at its core is a simple concept, is one that will be immensely helpful to your understanding, patience, and approach as your loved one becomes increasingly resistant to engage in outings and activities that he or she once enjoyed. I hope this lens also provides a peace through the confusion and disappointment of yet another good thing dementia seems to be taking away.

Prior to these new hesitations, other personality changes will undeniably occur. One of the most disruptive ones for both my dad and for those of us caring for him, has been his new tendency to constantly move things around. Since he can say, "No," but we as caregivers shouldn't tell them, "No," or "Don't," I've broached the topic by joking with him that this is a cruel trick that he's playing on himself since it's hard enough to remember where you put things even without dementia. At that, he has laughed, but he hasn't stopped this mind game he plays with himself. Unfortunately, he sometimes also plays it with others. One of the most notable and humorous instances of this was when my mom went out of town one day and came home to find that he'd mixed all of her well-labeled spices together in one big jar. And since most of these spices aren't common in grocery stores in the Midwest, it was a bigger "mix-up" than it seemed to be on the surface.

Moving things around is an obsessive behavior, stemming from his enjoyment of organizing. Another obsession that began forming before his dementia diagnosis, but then worsened with its onset and progression, centers around their yard. For a few years, he was consumed by the intent to make their yard perfectly flat and completely weed free. In this endeavor, he manually regraded over eighty percent of the yard and then started pulling "weeds" until there were no weeds or grass left. At the height of it, their address pulled up on Google maps showing half of the front yard stripped down to dirt and him knelt over pulling weeds in the background. Currently, there's a mixture of green grass and weed foliage in their mostly flat front yard, although the water meter has a retaining wall of sorts that dad built around it. Even to a fault, dementia has not broken my dad's exceptional work ethic.

He gets lost in his obsessions. He also loses track of time now. You're going to find that the person you're caring for will need to be reminded multiple times about time-sensitive events. While this can be frustrating for both the caregiver and for the loved one with dementia, I have to hope that this is because our loved ones are living in the moment and that it's a moment they're enjoying. I try to frame it as a unique form of mindfulness even in the absence of a fully-functioning mind.

Even when my dad's mind was fully functioning, he was not a characteristically warm personality. He was a good dad, offering his presence, his involvement, and his guidance. But his human irritability was often set off by a short internal fuse. Dementia has made this worse. It has also seemed to deteriorate the filter he did have between thought and word. With this, remaining as calm and as patient as I'd like to through some interactions is very challenging.

I've had many failed attempts at handling my dad's screaming or aggressiveness with grace. There have even been instances where I've thought to myself, "This is going to get stupid," with "this," being stupidity on my part for engaging in something that I knew wouldn't ultimately be worth it. Most recently, the stupidity revolved around an online video my dad found and was excitedly showing me. The video featured a couple of his favorite actors, lip-syncing and dancing to some of his favorite childhood songs. He was certain that they were the ones singing. I was certain they were not. He became upset, thinking I was minimalizing their talents. I became irritably dumbfounded that he couldn't tell that the voices didn't sound like theirs or that their lips didn't even always match up to the words being sung. I tried to explain that I could just as easily put a video of the late, great Whitney Houston on and lip-sync and dance around in their living room, but that wouldn't mean that I was singing or could ever sound like her. He conceded, but then he insisted that it was a couple of DJs singing, and that the actors were dancing. I tried to explain that even though the actors were dancing, DJs singing wasn't the case either. He would not believe it. He maintained that nobody was lip-syncing. We both double-downed until I finally listened to that voice in my head, that by then was laughing at me about how stupid it was to argue with him about this. By now, I'd already learned that correcting him was generally not effective, and in this case, it wasn't even important.

One of the least humorous and most heated examples of my falling from grace came during another visit to my parents' house in which I was there trying to help them. My dad had been especially combative all day, and I could no longer tolerate him yelling at my mom. Consequently, I completely lost my cool, stepped in between them, and yelled back at him that if he could yell, then I could yell louder. He upped his game, and I upped mine. I don't think either of us won that screaming match, but I did feel like a loser in reacting that way.

The next day, as I was sadly rehashing this to a friend who a few years prior had lost her mother to Alzheimer's Disease, I was reminded that I'm human and to give myself grace. Upon hanging up, I did. While I still wasn't proud of how I'd handled myself, I stopped beating myself up over it, understanding that I did the best I could in the moment and that I'd try to do even better the next time. As caregivers, that's all we can do, and it is enough.

Letting yourself make mistakes is very important in this journey. And finding a respect and forgiveness for yourself in knowing that you're showing up, even if imperfectly, is essential. Remind yourself that even if the care you're offering may feel like it's not "enough," it is one hundred percent better than not helping at all; and be proud of the assistance you are giving because it is vital. If you weren't showing up to care for your loved one with dementia, how horrendous would his or her situation be? It'd be exponentially worse than however badly you think you handled whatever tough interaction you just faced.

Through these and other negative interactions I've had, I've found a couple of winning strategies that I hope will help you if or as agitation and combative behaviors become the new or exaggerated normal demeanor for your loved one. When he or she starts screaming, do not match the tone. As my story just illustrated, it's extremely difficult to try to deescalate the situation when feeling like you or other caretakers are under unfair fire. However, the quickest way to not burn the whole household down is to lower your voice. This hasn't worked one hundred percent of the time, but it has often helped calm my dad down as his voice automatically lowered to more closely match mine. This has then helped me feel more composed.

Another highly effective technique that I've used is to tell my dad that I can't hear him when he yells. This is one of those times that tone is of the utmost importance. When I've tried to sarcastically say, "What? I can't hear you," he has picked up on the sarcasm and his agitation has increased. But when I've calmly stated that I can't hear him when he screams, the usual outcome is that he lowers his voice. This also lowers his agitation level to differing degrees.

Although combativeness and agitation are a normal part of the dementia journey, there's an important medical issue to check for when this behavior is excessive or sudden. It is a urinary tract infection. I'm not a doctor, so I'm not going to try to explain the correlation. However, I do know several people whose loved ones with dementia were experiencing urinary tract infections and displaying such uncharacteristic behaviors. Once the infections were treated, their behaviors adjusted back to whatever normal looked like at that point. This is an unexpected consideration, but keeping it in mind could be very helpful to you and to your loved one.

Along with these personality changes, you'll find that people with dementia become less grounded in current reality. The first time I experienced this was in my teenage years, volunteering at a nursing home. The lady I was visiting with was telling me about how her husband was going to pick her up for a dinner date. This sweet lady was bedridden, so I didn't understand how this was going to happen or why the nurse wasn't correcting her. As I saw her eyes sparkle talking about the dress she'd wear, my heart directed me to follow the nurse's lead and let her keep talking about it versus asking if she was sure this would happen. While I didn't know what I was witnessing at the time, or that it would ever be relevant in my life again, I know now why the nurse didn't stop her from indulging in this false expectation. It's natural to want to bring them back to reality in these moments, but when their thoughts or actions are not harmful, it's more effective and enjoyable to let go and to join them in their worlds.

To this end, we've found it beneficial in helping to curb some of the less desirable behaviors such as reorganizing things or landscaping, by encouraging other activities that my dad has liked in the past or is currently interested in. Effective tasks are often related to previous work or household functions or to recreational activities they once enjoyed. Another common thread amongst many people with dementia is the interest in music from their youth. It often helps to calm them down, to transport them to a place of clarity, and sometimes even to start a dance party. In fact, someone whose mother went to the adult day program with my dad recognized me on social media because he saw a picture of my dad. This caregiving son remembers my dad from doing the twist and starting his own dance party at the end of each day.

In execution, diving into his reality can be heart wrenching as I talk with my dad talk about dream vacations that I know he can no longer go on or see him turn everyday objects into toys. For Father's Day this year, part of his present was Play Dough, which he'd asked for to make an alien for a container he's painting to be a UFO. However, this is the side of getting to see him as he was as a child that makes me smile and illuminates the connection to the creativity and resourcefulness that I've known him to exhibit as an adult. Herein is a heartwarming solace.

CHAPTER 6:
ELVIS HAS LEFT THE BUILDING

"Memory loss is strange. It's like showing up for a movie after it's started. I'm sure I've missed something. I don't know if it's important or not. So I do the best I can to lose myself in the story and hope the gaps don't matter. Later, I can look it up, or someone will remind me, or maybe it's perfectly fine to not know."
Elizabeth Langston

Timelessly housed in an elegant gold frame, my favorite photo of my parents displays my then pregnant mom looking like a queen and my dad standing next to her looking like a king. This can partially be attributed to the beauty that youth naturally bestows. The other part is due to my dad proudly sporting the hairdo of a king. This king specifically is the King of Rock 'n' Roll, Elvis Presley.

Given my dad's affinity for all things music (music of his time that is, since his opinion is that modern music is "mostly garbage"), it's only natural that he's one of Elvis' biggest fans. As such, The King was impactful in the care my dad used to take in dressing and presenting himself with style. Now, this is another area in which dementia has affected his personality and habits.

Rather than dressing to the nines, Dad now dresses in a way that would be unstylish at any age or in any era. His style now is best described as comfort with a personal twist. This sounds acceptable, possibly even intriguing. In practice, it's that he rarely sees the value in changing out of fleece pants or elastic band shorts, either of those options often worn with an unmatching shirt.

The personal twist is executed and displayed through his sewing skills. He is convinced that all socks, even brand-new ones, need to have patches sewn onto the heels. As such, depending on the original reinforcement of the sock, certain pairs are now quite lumpy and uncomfortable. Rather than taking advice to stop sewing his socks (especially the pairs we've bought to replace the ones he has "customized"), he has instead crafted small pillows to address this discomfort. These pillows are similar to insoles, so the design makes sense from a conceptual standpoint. However, the logic stopped at theory because Dad's desire to sew didn't stop there. He'd wanted to take it a step further by sewing these pillows into his shoes. And just like the socks, he wanted to attach them regardless of the shoes' ages, conditions, brands, fits, or styles.

And the patches haven't stopped at socks. More visibly, he has started adding material to the ends of the arms and bodies of long sleeve sweatshirts, making them much too lengthy for his physique and resembling a child wearing an older sibling's clothes. To complete the custom look for each piece of an outfit, he got as far as sewing a small pillowy patch onto an awkward spot in the back of a pair of shorts, which added a "pouchy" look where there shouldn't be any bulk.

While the queen ruled against the "insoles" and the patched-up shorts, making sure my dad matches is no longer a battle my mom or I usually find worthwhile. However, an important change that dementia has caused related to this topic is one that we must address.

This shift is in regards to hygiene. A battle that we're still fighting revolves around getting my dad to change his clothes. Thankfully, he still is able and willing to shower every day, but from my research, I do know this is likely another impending change. We've tried laying out his clothes for him or offering to help him pick out clothes in an effort to increase his willingness to change his clothes by lowering his mental stress (since too many choices can be confusing to those with dementia). But neither of these methods have worked for us. However, these approaches have been successful for others so they'd be worth keeping in mind, should you have to cross this bridge. For appointments that pertain to him, I've been able to get him to change his clothes by noting that I've made the effort to be there for him, so he should also make the effort for himself. The success has come with his grumbles, but it has worked!

However, the most effective method for longer-term success with this for my dad has been getting him on a routine in which he does not feel pressured. During the months he was staying with me, we discussed how he could switch his showers to the nights and then change his clothes after the shower, not being asked to change again until after the next night's shower. I also made sure he knew that I would take care of washing his worn clothes so that he didn't run out. The agreement and reassurance are what seemed to hold the positive impact. He will be staying with me again in the upcoming months, so I'm hopeful we can ease back into this routine.

A couple other aspects of hygiene that are slowly degrading are his willingness to cut his nails and him remembering to shave each day. I've offered to cut his nails for him, but he won't allow it. Conversely, offering a reward sometimes encourages him to do it. As I mentioned in an earlier chapter, picking battles is an important measure towards keeping your peace. With this, I don't usually mention shaving to him, since he has not let it grow to a length where cleanliness would be of concern. But I will broach the topic with him on occasion, especially if it's bothering my mom. In those instances, I usually approach it with humor. One instance in which we were talking about it, and he knew he was being stubborn just for the sake of it, I joked that he used to take pride in his appearance, but now it seemed that Elvis had left the building. He laughed really hard and shaved the next morning. Dementia has taken some of his daily hygiene habits, but thankfully not his sense of humor.

Neither you nor your loved one with dementia will be able to stop or control these changes in dress and hygiene. This will likely frustrate you more than it will bother your loved one since he or she may not understand the importance of it. But understanding that these hygiene issues are a normal part of this abnormal process can help you more mindfully decipher which changes are a priority to contend with and which ones are safe to address with less frequency.

You may also find yourself at times taking an observational approach. A couple of the observations I've had are that even though my dad doesn't remember to shave, he still insists on and remembers to use Rogaine daily and that he will only go to his preferred barber (although his willingness to get his hair cut is also decreasing). From this point of detachment, I can see that although dementia doesn't produce runway styles, it also has not completely stolen my dad's sense of style. While Elvis might have left the building, The King still makes appearances.

CHAPTER 7:
IT'S ALSO ABOUT YOU

"You really have to love yourself to get anything done in this world."
Lucille Ball

"I'm listening to Linkin Park and trying not to drink." As I hovered alone over a puzzle that my dad and I had started a couple of weeks prior, this was my response to a check-in text from a friend one evening during the time that dad was staying with me. Her text came shortly after someone who is keenly aware of my heavy load had asked me if I would do something that could've much more seamlessly been taken care of by her. I had no emotional space or energy to give to this extraneous task. So while the angst-fueled song I was listening to was released more than twenty years before this night, it felt timely and appropriate for my current situation. This exchange was at the end of a day in which I'd cleaned up multiple accidents made by my parents' senior doggy and had bickered with my dad through most of those messes and accompanying clean-up. I was not proud of how I'd handled everything with him that day; but at least in that moment that night, my dad was contentedly watching television with their sweet dog sleeping next to him.

Earlier in that same day, I'd had a humorously defining revelation. Mom and I had recently convinced my dad to consider wearing absorbent underwear through the night so that should he need it in the future, he'd be used to it and could sleep better. Incontinence of differing forms and to differing degrees is another change that your loved one will likely encounter. My parents' dog's dementia made incontinence more of a challenge for her than dementia was making it for my dad. Nonetheless, him proactively agreeing to this type of undergarment was definitely a win. That afternoon, when I was in a big box store trying to find the right ones (the first time I'd faced this aisle alone), another customer was walking by shooting me a flirtatious look and about to strike up a conversation. Then he noticed the aisle I was in, meekly grinned, and very quickly walked away. In that moment, I could only laugh, as I thought to myself, "Hmm, so this is my life now."

And in this season of life, one of my biggest challenges has been that I've lost what I now know is the luxury of getting to be just a daughter. My parents have always been there for me, so to me, it's not an obligation, but an honor to get to be there for them now. I sometimes have guilt in wishing I weren't needed to the extent that I am, but if I weren't to fulfill this role, I would regret not caring for them in their time of need. However, from now being transportation provider, medical advocate, sporadic maintenance help, task runner, confidant, and IT advisor, I often don't have time or energy left to be their daughter in the same capacity as I was before the days of Dad's dementia. I mourn that role, and I'd love to have more moments of pure recreation with them.

As such, I'm currently exploring options to help me help them. One such resource that many communities have is a transportation service for senior citizens. These buses and vans usually provide low-cost door-to-door rides and come equipped with mobility features. My mom has not tried this yet, but my dad used it when he was going to the adult day program.

One of my friends from the support group told me that she was able to enjoy her mom more as a daughter again once she'd placed her in a care facility. I've also had another friend tell me that same thing; and she expanded that her dad became very ill when he was taking care of her mom who had Alzheimer's Disease. Her mom has passed away, but her dad is now in a nursing home since he can't recover from the health problems he incurred during his time as a caregiver.

This, along with helping my mom recover from the increasing health challenges she has been facing these past few years while caring for my dad, has alerted me to how important it is to not only take care of our loved ones with dementia, but to also watch out for our other aging parents. Residential placement is an effective option for some families, and adult day programs have been very helpful to my dad and to my mom and me in terms of socialization and keeping a routine for him and respite care for my mom and me. We are still trying to figure out the best solution long-term for our family, especially since the day program that my dad attended closed down amidst COVID-19 and has never reopened. After this closure is when my mom's health began declining more rapidly. Emotionally, this decline has brought about a separate heartache for me, and functionally, it has doubled my caregiving load and further lessened my opportunities to enjoy my parents as a daughter.

From a daughter to a caregiver, dementia has taught me that we cannot predict the future or our roles in it. However, I am certain that a change in living situation is imminent. To this end, we've discussed selling my parents' house and exploring options for them to move them in with us or live much closer to us in a way that would still allow everyone to have space and live comfortably. This could also allow Mom to safely have more respite from Dad. I envision something like a compound complete with a specially fenced-in area for my dad to pull weeds or grass! Joking aside, I reason that a couple of houses on the same plot of land or one big house with a couple of living spaces would not only be safer for them and make it easier for me to care for both of them, but it might also allow me to have more of those moments purely as their daughter. Our time together in this type of scenario would increase, so it couldn't be fully consumed with caretaking "to-dos," like it almost is now.

My acquaintance who recognized Dad from his dance parties has been caring for his mother in her home, with the help of a visiting caregiver agency. He recently contacted me stating that he's worried about the decline in his own health from taking care of her and is now facing the decision to place her in a home. I've never actually met either of them in person, but I can only guess that she wouldn't have wanted her son to decline along with her. Nonetheless, the internal struggle he is facing is a battle that shows no clear winner. In my reply to him on decision day I said, "I know we haven't met, but I'll be thinking of you both today." As you read this, if you're finding yourself in the same difficult decision-making space, I'd like to extend the same sentiment to you and your loved ones. It's a grueling journey with tough decisions, but you are not alone in it.

Like my acquaintance, my health has also suffered in this caregiving journey, albeit to a lesser degree than his or my mom's. As such, I'm learning the imperativeness of self-care. Just like my mom, caring for others comes naturally to me. But taking care of myself does not. However, I must. You must. If we deplete our reserves, we're increasingly likely to face caregiver burnout, other emotional distress, and physical problems.

I'm a believer in sharing light when others are in dark places. But this dementia-caregiving journey poses the real question of what might happen should your wick burnout.

What will happen to you? What will happen to those you care for?

With this in mind, begin rewiring any previous conditioning that framed self-care as selfish to the more accurate mindset that self-care is loving and necessary. Through behavior that replenishes you and brings you back to center, you actually have more to give your loved ones.

Take time and space to acknowledge and process the many emotions you're feeling and for doing things just for you, for your joy, for your preservation. Say, "No," when you need to. Get comfortable with, "No," becoming a complete sentence. Do all of this without guilt. I understand this is much easier typed than done, but this journey changes not just the people afflicted with dementia, but also their caregivers. If you do not make yourself a priority, you may find yourself in a position in which you are no longer able to take care of your loved one or yourself.

Self-care can take many different forms and will look and feel different on different days. Some days may not allow for even an hour of it, planned or unplanned, but don't let postponement turn into cancellation that ultimately manifests as damaging self-neglect. Whether it's napping, socializing, pursuing a hobby, exercising, getting a massage, watching television, doing absolutely nothing, or any other method you find effective to unplug and to reset, remind yourself that taking care of yourself is necessary. Reach out to someone or some group that can help you meet this need. This journey can feel very isolating, but there are people who want to help. As a caregiver to someone with dementia, self-care is survival for you and your loved one. Self-care will allow you to keep giving a care.

CHAPTER 8:
YET LOVE REMAINS

"Be where you are; otherwise, you will miss your life."
~Buddha

Dementia is often called the long goodbye. Our loved one is knowingly and unknowingly saying goodbye to memories, mental and physical functions, friends, experiences, independence, and personality. We, as caregivers, are also letting go.

We are letting go of our loved ones with dementia in a unique and painful way. Dementia forces us into a drawn-out grieving process, as we witness our loved ones losing these pieces of themselves little by little. They fight this loss, they debate with you through stages of it, unknowingly standing up for the thief that is this disease. And at times, they no longer fight the changes or fight you through the changes. In those moments, they succumb to a position where they wouldn't identify with who they once were or with who you know them to truly be.

The loss, the resistance, and the loss of resistance can all feel hopeless and infuriating. To offset these the negative feelings, it's helpful to keep in mind that your loved one with dementia isn't necessarily trying to give you a hard time, but is instead having a hard time. This important sentiment will help you approach your loved one with compassion and in a way that lets him or her know that (s)he is safe. In turn, this comfort you impart can restore a little bit of the power you feel dementia is taking away. Letting your loved one know that your words or actions come from a place of caring can work wonders in compliance. The compliance, or lack thereof, will differ from day to day and stage to stage.

There are many stages of dementia. Each one can vary in disruption to daily life and in length. It's daunting to have an idea of what's coming next but to not really know if or when it will. When it does, seeing these changes and not being able to stop them is a helpless feeling. But knowing what to expect can help ease these transitions, can add a feeling of normalcy to the abnormalities, and with the help of your loved one's medical team, can possibly deter some disease progression.

A medical specialist that will be important to find soon after diagnosis is a neurologist. This doctor will be able to help identify what stage your loved one is at and some of what can be expected during this time. You'll also be working closely with him or her to find and adjust medications and lifestyle to help slow disease progression down and manage symptoms as best as possible. Through testing and evaluations, the neurologist can also give you an educated judgement on which type or types of dementia your loved one is facing (Alzheimer's Disease is one form of dementia). This diagnosis will provide information on behavioral and caretaking expectations. At my dad's most recent neurology visit, my mom and I were thinking that his neurologist would determine at this appointment that he'd entered the next stage. I became even more certain of this when she asked him to stick out his tongue for the physical exam, and he timidly tried to decline, saying "That's bad!" and giggled in an uncharacteristically shy way. True to the twists and turns of dementia, he then ended up performing better on the recall test than he had the previous year! So even though dementia surfaces differently on different days and long-term prognosis is bad, that was a good day.

As it varies from day to day and sometimes hour to hour, dementia manifests differently for different people, so there's no one-size-fits-all solution; and there's no definitive way of knowing exactly how it will impact your loved one's life or your own. When I used to imagine what life would look like at my age, I pictured myriad things in addition to career aspirations. What I didn't picture was being this well-versed on dementia medicines and protocols. I also didn't envision that reality at this age would be friendships taking a backseat; constantly trying to help my parents, yet feeling helpless against dementia; and wistfully thinking that random places I'm driving by look like fun happy hour spots with coworkers, happy hours that I can't have right now since I've largely placed my career on hold to fulfill this important caregiving role.

So along with saying goodbye to my dad as I knew him, I've also been saying goodbye (or, "See you later,") to pieces of my identity. Despite losing these pieces of myself, I find a peace in knowing that my parents are well cared for and that I'm being as good of a daughter as I am able to be through these caregiving years. So, like my dad, I have also had to stop fighting what I thought life should look like, and I've gained the acceptance of allowing myself to be in this stage of life as it is now. Some days this acceptance comes easily, and other days I struggle with it and with the accompanying guilt of not wanting to succumb to it. However your caregiving years alter the shape of your life course, I hope you find a peace in this path that can only be realized through acceptance.

It has taken me years to come to this realization, but one morning I woke up with an enlightening acceptance of the fact that in this season, this is my job. I never imagined it would be at this stage of my life, and I wish this intense level of caregiving weren't necessary (for my family or for yours). But since this is my new normal, I now can't imagine not fulfilling this caregiving role that's fueled and renumerated by love. And in the end, with all that dementia takes from our loved ones and from us, it cannot take away the love or the care that's shared between us.

"What counts in life is not the mere fact that we have lived. It is what difference we have made to the lives of others that will determine the significance of the life we lead."
Nelson Mandela

ABOUT THE AUTHOR

Pratibha Vanmali graduated high school from a rural Midwest town and furthered her education as a Churchill Scholar at Westminster College in Fulton, Missouri. While in school, she explored creative opportunities in writing, graphic design, and photography and has employed what she learned through those avenues in work, volunteerism, and play since graduating.

Her sincerity and passion are evidenced in her work. And her love of travel, combined with her artistic nature, have allowed her to write and shoot nationally and internationally, being published in award-winning magazines and working with clients who have been featured on Oprah, Jay Leno, ESPN, Ellen DeGeneres, and Pet Stars.

You are impressively resilient.

Pratibha

You're doing a great job.

Madhuben
(Pratibha's Mom)

You're due for self-care.

Pratibha

Inhale. Smile. Exhale.

♡

Pratibha

My Companion Has Dementia and Might Have Difficulty Communicating.

We Appreciate Your Patience and Kindness.

Hello, I'm

_______________________.

I Have Dementia.
My Emergency Contact Is:

_______________________.